EATING YOUR WAY TO A BETTER HEALTH

A Guide to Healthful eating

By

Evan I. Curtis

TABLE OF CONTENTS

Chapter 1

Introduction to Healthful eating

Chapter 2

Understanding micronutrients and micro nutrients

Chapter 3

Planning a Balanced Meal

Chapter 4

Eating Healthy on a Budget

Chapter 5

Understanding Food Allergies And Intolerance

Chapter 1

Introduction to Healthful eating

Healthful eating is a way of life that focuses on making mindful food choices that nourish the body and promote overall health. Eating healthfully doesn't have to be complicated or boring. It's all about being aware of the nutritional value of the food you're consuming, and making choices that are beneficial to your health and wellness. Healthful eating involves selecting a variety of nutrient-dense foods, such as lean proteins, fresh fruits and vegetables, whole grains, legumes, and healthy fats. Eating healthfully also includes limiting processed foods, reducing added sugars and saturated fats, and drinking plenty of water. Making healthful choices can help you maintain a healthy weight, reduce your risk of certain chronic diseases, and provide you with the energy you need to live an active lifestyle.

Healthful eating is not a one-size-fits-all approach; it's important to recognize that everyone's nutritional needs are different. Working with a registered dietitian can help you create an individualized meal plan that meets your specific needs. With the right guidance, you can learn to make healthful food choices that are both enjoyable and nutritious.

With a few simple steps, you can start your journey towards healthful eating today. Start by familiarizing yourself with the basics of nutrition and making small changes to your diet. Choose nutrient-dense foods, read labels, plan meals and snacks, and get creative in the kitchen. With the right tools, you can make healthful

eating an enjoyable and
sustainable part of your life.

Happy eating!

Chapter 2

Understanding macronutrients and micronutrients

Macronutrients are nutrients that the body needs in large amounts to function properly. They include proteins, carbohydrates, and fats. Each of these macronutrients provides either energy or structural support to the body.

Proteins are made up of amino acids and are used for growth and repair of the body's tissues. Carbohydrates provide energy for the body's cells and are found in grains, fruits, vegetables, and other foods. Fats provide energy and also help with the absorption of some vitamins and minerals.

Micronutrients are nutrients that the body needs in smaller amounts, but are still important for health. These include vitamins, minerals, and phytochemicals (chemicals found in plants).

Vitamins and minerals help the body to function properly by regulating various metabolic processes, while phytochemicals are thought to provide health benefits.

While this nutrients are important for good health, it is important to remember that they should be consumed in the right amounts. Eating too much or too little of any nutrient can lead to health problems. In general, a balanced diet with a variety of foods from all food groups should provide all the

nutrients that the body needs.

In conclusion, macronutrients and micronutrients are both essential for good health. Eating a balanced diet with foods from all food groups will ensure that the body gets the right amount of each nutrient.

Chapter 3

Planning a Balanced Meal

Planning a balanced meal is an essential part of a healthy lifestyle.

 A balanced meal can provide the body with the essential nutrients, vitamins, and minerals it needs to maintain good health. Eating a balanced meal can help to reduce the risk of obesity, heart disease, and other health conditions.

 A balanced meal should include a variety of foods from all of the food groups.

Each of these food groups provides different nutrients, vitamins, and minerals that the body needs for proper functioning. The main food groups are grains, vegetables, fruits, dairy, and protein. Eating a variety of foods from each group can help to ensure that the body is getting the necessary nutrients.

 Here are some tips for planning a balanced meal:

1. Start with a variety of colorful fruits and vegetables: Choose both fresh and frozen options that are rich in vitamins and minerals.

 2. Include whole grains: Try to include whole grains such as quinoa, millet, oats, and brown rice.

3. Include lean proteins: Lean proteins such as poultry, fish, beans, and legumes are good sources of essential amino acids.

4. Include healthy fats: Healthy fats such as avocados, nuts, and seeds are important for maintaining good health.

Chapter 4

Eating Healthy on a Budget

Eating healthy on a budget can be challenging, but it is possible with a little planning and creativity. To start, make a shopping list of the items you need to buy. Stick to the list and avoid impulse purchases. Look for sales and discounts at the grocery store, and buy generic brands if available. Consider shopping at bulk stores, farmer's markets, and ethnic specialty stores for better prices.

Prepare meals at home instead of eating out. Plan your meals ahead of time and make a grocery list accordingly. Look for ways to get creative with ingredients, such as using a variety of vegetables, beans, and grains. Prepare meals in bulk and freeze single-serving portions for later.

Learn how to cook basic meals and experiment with a variety of healthy recipes. Use a slow cooker or pressure cooker for easy meals that require little effort. Make use of leftovers and create new dishes with what you have on hand.

Choose nutrient-dense, whole foods to get the most nutrition for your money.

Stock up on frozen vegetables, canned fish, beans, and other healthy staples. Avoid processed foods, which are often more expensive and contain unhealthy ingredients.

Make healthy snacks ahead of time, such as energy bars, trail mix, or yogurt with granola. Eat healthy snacks can help you avoid cravings for unhealthy foods.

Finally, stay hydrated by drinking plenty of water.

Avoid sugary drinks and opt
for herbal teas instead.

Eating healthy on a budget is
possible if you take the time
to plan ahead and shop
smart. With a little effort,
you can make healthy meals
that are both delicious and
affordable.

Chapter 5

Understanding Food Allergies And Intolerance

Food allergies and intolerance are two different conditions that are often confused. While both can cause uncomfortable symptoms, they are caused by different reactions within the body.

A food allergy occurs when the body's immune system mistakes a food protein for a harmful substance and produces antibodies to fight it. This can cause a range of symptoms including hives, swelling, vomiting, and difficulty breathing. These reactions can be life-threatening and require immediate medical attention.

Food intolerance, on the other hand, occurs when

the digestive system has difficulty breaking down a certain food. Common symptoms of food intolerance include abdominal pain, bloating, gas, and diarrhea. Unlike food allergies, food intolerance reactions are not life-threatening.

It's important to understand the difference between food allergies and intolerance so that you can take the necessary steps to prevent or manage them correctly. If you suspect you may have a food allergy or intolerance, it's important to speak to your doctor for a proper diagnosis.

The best way to avoid a food allergy or intolerance reaction is to avoid the food completely. However, if that's not possible, there are several steps you can take to minimize your risk. These include taking an antihistamine to reduce the severity of symptoms, eating small portions of the food, and checking food labels for potential allergens.

Finally, it's important to be aware of the signs of a food allergy or intolerance reaction and to get medical help if needed. Symptoms can range from mild to severe, and prompt treatment is the best way to avoid a serious reaction.

Understanding food allergies and intolerance can help you

take the necessary steps to ensure your safety and well-being.

In conclusion, Eating Your Way to a Better Health has provided an abundance of useful information on healthful eating. We have explored the benefits of a well-balanced diet, the importance of portion control, and the variety of healthy foods available. We have discussed the importance of mindful eating and have provided tips on how to make healthy choices when eating out.

Eating Your Way to a Better Health has provided you with the tools you need to make informed food choices. Now that you have the knowledge, it's up to you to put it into action and make small changes to your diet.

With these simple steps, you can make a big difference in

your overall health and
wellbeing.

www.ingramcontent.com/pod-product-compliance
Lightning Source LLC
Chambersburg PA
CBHW061550250726

48657CB00006B/2411